Kettlebell Workouts For Beginners:

Essential Kettlebell Exercises to Build Strong Muscles and Have a Healthy Body

By

Paul Keithley

ISBN-13: 978-1508624158

Table of Contents

Kettlebell Workouts For Beginners: Essential Kettlebell Exercises to Build Strong Muscles and Have a Healthy Body

By Paul Keithley

Introduction

The kettlebells have been used in many centuries for ballistic training by athletes. They have become the ultimate forms of exercises since they work out all the muscles of the body at once. The bells are effective mostly for strengthening and flexing the muscles of the body, from the toes to the upper part of the body. There are different techniques that are meant to have effect on different body muscles. Most of the professional trainers in the world have adopted the use of the kettlebells to keep their players in form by strengthening their muscles. However, the use of this training kits should be done in a professional way to avoid injuries. This is however mostly in the case of beginners. By the end of this book, you will progress to the more skilled level and not just the beginner.

Chapter 1. Principles of Kettlebell Training

The use of the kettlebells requires the use of different principles before effective changes can be experienced in the body of the athlete (or any other trainee for that matter). The different principles are meant to achieve different effects on different body muscles. Before you embark on any of the training principles, you need to be certain that it is the most effective one. You can also seek the guidance of a professional trainer who will guide you on which technique to use and how often to apply it. Here are some of the most common principles of kettlebell training;

a) The kettlebell squatting- This is one of the most common techniques used in training by use of the kettlebells. The muscles of the knee are the most effected on this technique. The other muscles that are involved on this technique include the thigh muscles, the hips and the buttocks. This technique can use two kettlebells or one depending on the instructions given by the trainer.

One of the things to keep in mind when doing the kettlebell squatting technique is that when you squat, your back should always be in a straight position. Well, you can always start with simple steps to achieve this. The next step is usually to lift the kettlebell.

There are different variations through which you can do the squat lifting. The most common variations are the goblet squat and the double squat. The end results of the two variations is usually the same although they vary in position of the kettlebell.

b) The Kettlebell lunge- As much as this principle involves the knee, the buttocks are the most effected one. The technique is being used by many personal trainers all over the world due to its effectiveness. In this technique, the chest should always be up and straight. When performing this technique, one knee should always be nearly touching the floor and both knees should be in a 90° position. Stability may be a problem at first but you will get used to it as you progress with the training. Just like the kettlebell squat technique, you can employ the use of two kettlebells on each hands or one kettlebell. To make this effective, always pass the kettlebell under your feet to the opposite side.

c) The kettlebell deadlift

This is also a common principle that beginners can use to build the muscles of the body. It is an easy technique that has massive positive in building the strength of different muscles on the body of the athletes and trainees in general.

Always stand upright with the kettlebell between your legs. You will then bend from your hips and lift the kettlebell. Make sure that your back is in a parallel position with the ground and that your posterior shin is vertical. All this precautions are to maximise the effects the technique will have on the muscles. The shoulders should be held straight up when lifting the kettlebell. One precaution to keep in mind is that the kettlebell should not just be listed up straight from the ground. It should be done in a pulling manner on the ground way up. Squeeze your gluteus muscles as you lift the kettlebell off the ground. On returning it, make sure that it is at the spot that you took it from in the ground. This helps in self-adjusting the muscles.

The buttocks and the hamstring are the most strengthened muscles on this technique. The back and core muscles are also affected by this technique.

d) The kettlebell swing

This technique usually utilises the same principle that the kettlebell deadlift uses. As a beginner seeking to use this technique, you can start with all the instructions that are on the kettlebell deadlift but during the lifting time, the ball should be hiked between your legs.

After you have bent like in the deadlift position, you will then reach out for the kettlebell. There is the kettlebell back swing and the kettlebell upswing variations. The backswing requires more force and you should be prepared to use some more energy. The ball should then be returned to its starting position. You can perform 10 swings to get the best results from the same principle. The back and thigh muscles are usually the most involved on this principle. This technique can be most effective especially if you employ the use of a trainer, a professional one for that matter.

Chapter 2. Kettlebell Workouts

To achieve effective results from the use of the kettlebells, you need to keep in mind the workouts and the exercises that you are required to follow up. Failure to follow the laid down workout procedure will eventually lead to undesired results. In order for you to progress, you have to do it right. You can always employ the skills and advice of a professional trainer who will get you through this program. Let us take you through the kettlebell training program that you need to follow up to achieve the best results. There are some key factors that you need to put in mind before you can have a successful training program.

1. Well, before you start any workout, keep in mind to always start with the kettlebell strength exercises rather than doing conditioning ones. This is to reduce the chances of you getting fatigued and legs being shaky. When you are fatigued, you will not be able to start the main workout program of the kettlebells.

2. You will have to be persistence when doing the program. Any athlete will tell you that to experience any changes in your body muscles, the training and workouts should be consistence. It does not necessarily mean that you train 5000 continuous hours. Kettlebells come in different weights and you have to progress from one weight to another and not to skip from 10kg to 24kg just because you need to see some changes in your muscle strength.

3. Work on your posture as you continue advancing the weights of the kettlebells that you lift. Never rush to see the changes in your body muscles. A trainer will always tell you that you need to start small so that your body muscles get used to the weights as they increase. This reduces the chances of you being hurt as you lift the weights. Adjustment of the muscles is also a good way of ensuring that the workout is successful at the end of the whole procedure.

4. You also need to know the muscles that will be affected with each of the kettlebell technique that you employ. Is there a point of doing a workout yet you do not know what effects it will have on your body? As we saw earlier,

the different techniques come with different body changes. Employing the right technique will see to it that you get you desired results. Still on this factor, always make sure that you use the techniques that will have effect on the whole body muscles. There is a difference between an athlete training and a normal training program.

5. Never employ all the techniques that you know in a single workout session. Sometimes people what to experience changes in their body strength and muscles and end up trying to achieve that in a single session. Always start with a single technique on each session, master it and get to see the effects that it has on your body. There are many techniques that you can employ. As the saying goes, Rome was never build on a single day, neither will the training programs. It is a common practise that men tend to go for the heavier weights unlike the women who tend to progress as he time goes. The main objective for any training is that you will gradually feel the changes on your body.

6. Keep your budget on the safe side when you are doing the workouts. Have you seen people that spend all they

have on workouts and end up going broke, only to not finishing the whole training course.

7. Do training and workouts that you are comfortable with. This goes hand in hand with the point of progressing on the weights that you lift. Sometimes you may end up lifting weights that are beyond you capabilities and you end up inflicting more injuries to yourself. This calls for the use of an experienced trainer who will see to it that you follow the procedures correctly.

The purpose of the training workouts is to be fit and also string. You have to be lift at least double 48kg kettlebells to be strong on the workout sessions. If you cannot do a single swing of 48kg for 20 minutes continuously, then are not strong and equally not fit.

In conclusion of the factors to consider before going on any workout program, try and use common sense. It comes in handy when you are doing the lifting. This also makes your progress be significant.

Chapter 3. How Long Should The Workouts Take?

The training programs using the kettlebell lifts usually varies depending on the effects that you want. Well, we will give you the best training program that will give you the best results. If you have your own kettlebells at home, then you do not have to go to the gym. The program will see to it that you get the best strength and fitness in your body. With the employment of the best techniques, be sure that you will experience the best and desired changes in your body strength. Training comes with many factors such as the nutrition and the time each workout will be taking. Once you follow the laid down procedures, you will not have any issues with the kettlebell training.

A typical training session can take about 30 minutes, 45 minutes or a whole hour. In the case of beginners, always start with 30 minutes so that you progress as your body adjusts to the weights. You do not want to overwork yourself when in training so that you give up within a short time. There are also some techniques that require less time than others. The desired effects that you want to get from the lifts also depends on the time that you take on each session. This is not to dispute the facts that all beginners should start slow and gradually increase the time as they adjust to the program.

Chapter 4. How Often to Exercise?

This is one area that tends to confuse lots of people and trainees in general. For how many days per week should you carry out the workout program?

This is one area that mostly depends on the schedule of the trainee. As a beginner, you can start with 3 days on the first weeks. This can be gradually increased to more days depending on how tight your schedule is. If you have more time, you can always do the kettlebell training for up to four days in week. This can be typically on Monday, Tuesdays, Thursday and Fridays.

Sometimes training for more days leads to more results. However, as a beginner, always start with fewer days on the first weeks so that your body can adjust on the different weights. You do not want to fatigue your body even before you have done all the training techniques.

You should also be certain on the times that you rest. Well, our bodies are not machines that operate throughout. You will need to strategies on the times that you will be resting between each circuit and also which days you should be resting in the week. The more rest your body gets, the better for the muscles. Your body and health will play a major part in you strategizing the time that you require for resting. One other reason that you need to rest more is that just in case you have an injury, it will heal perfectly.

One of the major that you need to keep in mind in this training sessions and plans is that you should never miss one. The moment you start skipping one, then your whole program will go down in shatters and you will not achieve what you have been looking for. Try as much as possible to stick to the laid down plans and trust me, you will get the desired results without much hustle. Many trainees have backed down on the kettlebell training programme since they have not been following the procedures.

During the workout sessions, you may encounter a technique that you know nothing about. Never worry, as long as you have read the above techniques, you will be more than ready to do it. Your trainer will also assist at this point. Never try to force a technique lest you inflict more injuries on yourself.

Chapter 5. The Best Kettlebell Training Plan For Beginners

We are going to take you through the best plans that you can use to get the best results in the kettlebell training program. Before you can start on any program, always make sure that you have the necessarily equipment's, that is, a kettlebell or two and some appropriate gear.

WEEK ONE

Session 1

The first week is usually most crucial since the beginners body has not yet adopted to the systems and the lifts.

The first session will involve warm up training such as body weight squat, doing some arm circles (forward, large, backwards and small). This is to prepare the body to be fit when you start the lifting techniques using the kettlebells. The warm up exercises should not be extreme to the extent that they fatigue your body.

After you have warmed up, you can start with some kettlebell front squat technique. You can start with 3 rounds of 30, 20 and 10 of each technique that we have discussed above. You can always start with small rounds if you feel that you may be exhausted at some point.

On the first workout, you can also complete 20 rounds of kettlebell swings and also dead lift. This will prepare your muscles for even harder sessions and lifts. The rest period should be 30 seconds before you shift to the next technique. This gives the grace period for the muscles to return to the original position. You should never make mistake of resting for longer times lest the muscles over relax. You can complete this session with five push-ups and the first session will be done.

b) Session 2

This session also requires you to do some warm ups and you will be ready to go. The warm ups this time will involve back slaps, trunk rotations, steam engine and the BW squat. You will take the front squat technique on this level during the training session. The push press can also be done on this level. All the techniques that are done on this session are done six times each having 60 seconds.

You can also use other kettlebell lifting principles on this session so that your body muscles start to adopt.

c) Session 3

Make sure that you do the same warm ups that you did on the second session. The training programme on this session involves the front squatting, high pull and the kettlebell swing. You will also do the weighted sit-up 15 times. Be sure that your muscles will hurt at some point on this session especially of you did not do enough warm ups. The resting time before the next training will remain 60 seconds.

d) Session 4

Start with small warm up sessions of 3 round each on push-ups, 10 times on steam engine and 20 times on the jumping jack. Training on this session also involves the use of different kettlebell techniques. The kettlebell lunge can be done 10 times for three rounds. This should involve each leg having its own 3 rounds. The next technique that should be done after 60 seconds should be lunge cycle which should be done five times.

The iso squat should be done for 60 seconds on this training session. The beginner trainee should also do 3 rounds of kettlebell deadlift, 10 times of chest press and 20 times of front squat. This point requires that you do the same for 15 minutes each.

Session 5

In the warm up part of this session, you will perform 10 kettlebell swings and 5 times on the kettlebell lounge. You can also add five times of weighted sit-ups. The training on this case requires more strength and dedication. At this stage, you are no longer a beginner and you have the perfect skill that is required to do even more training. Each of the technique that is done on this training session is done four times.

Session 6

You will also do warm ups on this session, just like in its predecessor session. Training is more complex than in session 5. In this session, the rounds of lifts that are to be performed are in the range of 25, 20, 15, 10 and a minimum of 5. The techniques that can be performed on this point include the kettlebell swing, weighted sit-up, the deadlift-high pull and the kettlebell twist. The resting times between each technique can vary between 30 and 60 seconds.

Session 7

The warm ups on this session are done for three rounds. You will perform the kettlebell lunge five times for each round. The bodyweight squat is also done 10 times for each round. The other warm up exercises that you can do on this session include trunk rotation and the alternate lunge. The training programme requires that you do 10 rounds of push press, half moon, front squat, kettlebell twist, Push press Right arm and the push press Left arm. You can also add two rounds of kettlebell deadlift which should be done twelve times each round, 24 times deadlift-high pull, 12 times kettlebell high pull and another 24 times of deadlift-high pull on each round. The time rest between the training techniques should be kept at 30 seconds.

Session 8

The warm up session here will involve 3 rounds of bodyweight squat and 30 push-ups. When you have reached this point in your training, then you are becoming a pro and your muscles will start showing significant changes. The actual training programs on this session will involve six rounds of 60 seconds each. The kettlebell techniques that are on this session include body

Session 9

You also need to warm up before you can start the training on this session. The warm up exercises include kettlebell swing, jumping jack and kettlebell twist. The training programmes that you will do in this case will involve 20 rounds. The techniques that you will practise include switching kettlebell swing, switching dead-high pull, half-moon and the weighted sit-up. You have to be persistent and complete all the 20 rounds.

Session 10

Each warm up on this session should be done for five rounds each. You can begin with the kettlebell lunge, then head to the steam engine for 30 seconds, the bodyweight squat for 30 seconds before you finish with the sit ups. The training that you will experience in this session should be done for 20 minutes each. You can begin with the front squat, half-moon, thruster, halo and the kettlebell swing.

Session 11

The warm ups should be done for three rounds each. Each round should involve five times per round for lunge, 10 times for bodyweight, 10 times for front squat and 5 times for jump start. Training should involve six rounds of 60 seconds each beginning with the kettlebell swing, switching swing, another round of the kettlebell swing, the overhead swing and the figure 8 pass through. You can rest for 30 seconds after each technique that you do on this session.

Session 12

The warm up section on this program is quite involving since you will do the kettlebell swing for 15 times. The weighted sit up right arm is done for five time as a warm up. You will complete with 10 push-ups and 5 weighted sit up on the left arm. The training techniques are done for 6 rounds, 2 minutes each and 30 seconds rest interval. In training, you will start with the thruster followed by the switching deadlift-high pull.

Session 13

The warm ups are also done for three rounds, 20 times for the deadlift, 10 times for the high pull, 20 times front squat and 10 push press. The training program involves Planck row on each arm, the deadlift high pull, weighted sit up, thruster and the standing chest press. You can finish with the overhead swing.

Conclusion

In conclusion, the kettlebell workouts for the beginners can be effective especially when you follow the laid down procedures and training programs. As we said before, skipping any of the program will lead to less significant results and that is why you should hire a trainer that will also guide you through the workout program. Trainees should also keep in mind their nutrition so that they do not end up losing your shape. Keeping a good nutrition will also see to it that you are gaining more muscles. Following this program to the latte will also see to it that you see the points that you need to correct and the muscles that need more training on. Kettlebell come in different weights and you should progress from the first week as you also gradually increase the weights. You do not want to skip to a higher weight just because you want to see the effects of the workouts immediately.

If you are not very sure about what techniques to use, then you need to consult the services of a trained professional who will guide you on the best techniques and workouts to use. Athletes always follow a workout procedure that guides them on how to do effective training. Always know that as a beginner, you have to start on small workout programs before you can proceed to the more advanced training programs. This may take a while but it is worth the wait. Patience pays. Also keep in minds that the warm ups will play a vital role in ensuring that you have the best workout procedures. Warming up ensures that the muscles are up active and that they can now begin handling muscles of different weights. The different warming up exercises that we have reviewed prepare different muscles for different techniques. Beginners are also advised to take rests between the techniques. This prepares the muscles so that you can shift to the next technique with easy. You can purchase your own kettlebell or visit the gym and use some that they have. If you have one in your home, then it will be easier follow the training program. You can use the manual that we have provided for you and will experience drastic changes in your body shape. Your muscles will never hurt after you have employed the use of the different techniques.

Thank You Page

I want to personally thank you for reading my book. I hope you found information in this book useful and I would be very grateful if you could leave your honest review about this book. I certainly want to thank you in advance for doing this.

If you have the time, you can check my other books too.

www.ingramcontent.com/pod-product-compliance
Lightning Source LLC
Chambersburg PA
CBHW071345310526
45790CB00018B/1367